Poems

for

Medical Students

by

Cate Chason

10 9 8 7 6 5 4 3 2 1

ISBN: 978-0-692-02156-9

Library of Congress Control Number: 2014937857

Chason, Cate
    Poems for Medical Students

1. Poetry. I. Title

Printed in the U.S.A. by Des Printing
Cover photo: Cate Chason
Cover design, editing and layout: Jill Culora, Husking Bee Art & Media

I dedicate this book to Lillian, and her astonishing sister, Hannah Morgan Chason if for no other reason than to hear the two words Lillian and Hannah in the same breath, over and over.

Lillian's Legacy

The news from Mya, our daughter, was at first unremarkable - Lillian was sick with the flu. As a pulmonologist, I was
seeing lots of influenza cases that fall. Almost all, without
exception, were of a mild form. Even though I knew the dire
warnings of this new strain, H1N1, I didn't give Lillian's illness
much thought.

A day later however, Eric called from North Carolina. Lillian was gravely ill. She was on a ventilator and in the ICU.
My heart sank.

In a split second, I stopped being a friend and assumed
the clinical detachment of a physician. Patients do die from
influenza, some 250,000 worldwide. Yes, lung involvement is a
serious concern. And yes, the young and the elderly are most
vulnerable.

But Lillian was at an excellent medical center, and I was
sure her doctors were treating her properly. This was 2009 after all, not the 1918 pandemic. Lillian would beat this. She was
a fighter, a life force. And as a doctor, I considered the facts,
and determined that all would be well.

Nonetheless I was also a parent and a friend. Oh my god,
I thought. Lillian could die. She really could die. Why is this
happening? Lillian must be so scared. How dreadful for Eric
and Cate and Hannah. Bad things can happen to good people.
Hadn't my own father been killed in a plane crash when I was

nine?! Just as improbable, Lillian could die from H1N1.

I fought my fears and promised Eric that I would catch a plane the next morning to North Carolina. I had to be part of the medical team and I wanted to be there for my friends.

At the hospital, Eric introduced me to the head physician, Anthony Charles. He showed me Lillian's chest x-ray. The radiograph should have been black. Yet it was densely white, indicating the airspaces were completely flooded with fluid. In all my years of practice, I had never seen such a lack of air in the lungs. In a drastic intervention, Lillian had been placed on ECMO (extracorporeal membrane oxygenation), a radical lifesaving machine which removes the blood, oxygenates it, and then recirculates it back into the body.

Feeling impotent, empty, angry, and afraid, I refused to fully accept that Lillian's chance of survival was slim and that my own expertise was unlikely to affect her medical outcome.

Over the next several weeks, we all traveled the ups and downs of her care. There were times of great hope as she inched closer to improvement and then the set backs, the worsening numbers, the complications. We all knew her time on ECMO was finite. We saw the grains of sand falling. So I danced as fast as I could: exploring Lillian's newest medical data with Eric, hugging Hannah, sharing with Cate the latest entries on the "Prayers for Lillian" website, and giving gentle words and soft touch to Lillian. How difficult and privileged to be on the edge of both worlds.

I had just returned home when Eric called to inform me that Lillian had passed away. I wasn't surprised but I cried. I cried for Lillian, for the Chasons, and for everyone who has ever lost someone special, including myself.

Lillian is with me every day in the hospital; when I take time to hold a patient's hand or answer another question from a family member. I feel her presence telling me to be more human, not just a purveyor of medical facts. I find comfort in knowing that Lillian lives on in Cate's poems and the every day remembrances that we all carry with us.

Chuck Sherman, MD
July 10, 2012
Providence, RI

If silence creates
reunion, I will shut my
endless screaming heart

One Month And One Day

On Sunday, November 15, 2009, our daughter Lillian sent us a text that said she was getting sick. One month and one day later, we had to tell the doctors it was okay to turn off her life support.

It started as a headache, with the doctor saying she was probably getting the flu. It progressed to acute respiratory distress syndrome and she spent three weeks on a machine, which replaced the function of her lungs, before we had to give up.

Lillian was a freshman at the University of North Carolina in Chapel Hill when she got sick. She had only been there for 10 weeks. In that time, she went through many of the difficulties of all freshmen ("Why isn't anyone asking me out?") but in general things were going well. Her main passion was acting and she had just won the lead role in a new play written by one of her professors. As she told her mother: "This place is perfect."

This statement was even more remarkable because Lillian was going blind. When she turned 16, we learned that she had a genetic form of macular degeneration that slowly destroys the central portion of the field of vision. There had been telltale signs before hand – trouble with eyeglass prescriptions, no longer able to catch fly balls – but it took a trip to the Mass

Eye and Ear Infirmary in Boston to confirm it.

After a long day of tests, the doctor came in to speak with us. He pulled his rolling stool up to where Lil was sitting so he would be at her level. She sat on her hands on the edge of the exam table, leaning forward, looking down at the floor.

"I'm sorry to be the person to tell you this, but you have Stargardt's disease. Your eyesight is going to keep getting worse. There's nothing that can be done about it."

She bit on her bottom lip, gently nodding her head and rocking her body. Then she put her hand on his knee and said "I understand. It's okay." He surprised us by turning away from her, trying to hide the tears forming in his eyes.

In her senior year of high school, she spent long hours working on her homework because it was getting harder and harder to read. She would stay up late into the night listening to her assignments on a special audiobook reader, wearing a large pair of headphones while she sat in her bed and knitted to maintain her concentration. Her physics and math assignments had to be magnified to large proportions. Their large text made them look like children's books but the content was college-level. She refused to drop behind, determined to prove that she was just as smart as anyone else. She wouldn't accept any less of herself just because she couldn't see.

And whenever she went out, she wore sunglasses. Some studies showed that exposure to sunlight accelerated the degeneration, so this was one of the few things we could do that might help. She had a great collection – her mother and I could never pass a Sunglass Hut without stopping in. Even the best were only a tiny way for us to compensate for all the things that she wouldn't be able to do, like driving a car.

She chose to go to the University of North Carolina in Chapel Hill, like her mother and a large contingent of uncles, aunts and cousins stretching back as far as memory served (which for a Southern family is pretty long). Lillian wanted to get away from the high pressure of the Northeast, where smart young women are made to feel like one-of-a-million instead of one-in-a-million. Old friends and family in the area opened their arms and homes to her, offering her any help she needed to get accommodated. We felt like she was in good shape when we drove away from her dorm that August. She waved us goodbye wearing her flip-flops and sunglasses, seeming perfectly ready for her new life at college.

Two weeks before Thanksgiving, Lillian called us to ask for the number of the university's retinologist. She had a stabbing pain behind her eyes and was panicked that she might be going blind more quickly than we'd anticipated. After examining her, the retinologist said her eyes were okay but that she was probably getting the flu. The next day, she went to student health services, where the doctor told her to go back to her dorm and try to get better.

"You're symptons will probably get worse," he said. "Don't worry and don't come back for a few days."

My wife wanted to fly down and help, but Lillian said she could take care of herself. She begged her to go back to the doctor, but Lillian insisted that he told her not to return yet. After two more days of phone calls and worrying, my now-frantic wife called her cousin who lived nearby and asked her to check up on her. By then Lillian was nearly in shock, and had to be taken directly to the emergency room.

The next morning, when my wife and I were finally able to reach North Carolina, Lillian was on a ventilator and her lungs were filling with fluid. The probable diagnosis was H1N1. After two more days, the doctors put her on a machine (known by its acronym ECMO) that oxygenated her blood and allowed her lungs to rest.

The story of her illness is beyond retelling here. It was an epic battle between the healing processes in her lungs and the complications induced by the life-supporting ECMO machine. One of her professors started a Facebook page for her called "prayersforlillian." In the three weeks Lillian spent in the hospital more than 10,000 people joined it, forming a virtual community hoping and praying for her to get better. She was on the machine for 23 days, but ultimately her lungs weren't able to recover quickly enough and she died on Dec. 16.

The day after Lillian died, we went to her dorm room to pack up her belongings before returning to Rhode Island for the funeral. The room was familiar to us. We had spent several days with her during orientation, making multiple treks to the surrounding stores to provide what we thought would make her comfortable. Yet, after living at the hospital for the last few weeks, it was shocking to be suddenly transported back into her world, surrounded by the objects of a life she was enjoying so much, a life that she would never resume.

In her closet I found her collection of sunglasses. Each case held its own world of memories, reminding me of when we bought them and of the girl who wore them. Of when her boyfriend, always protective of her, asked if it was okay when she took them off to be photographed for her senior prom. Of the girl with the Audrey Hepburn smile who wanted to be an actress and was selected to be the lead in her first college play. And of the sad realization that we had thought her failing eye-sight was going to be her big challenge in life—not realizing that we were the ones who were blind.

Eric Chason
March 3, 2013
Barrington, RI

Right With The World

Not long ago all felt right with the world
and I remember it.

In September
after returning from Chapel Hill

many times people asked
what is it like being an empty nester?

My reply was, how can I feel sad
when Hannah and Lillian are out there

thriving young women who will someday
make the world a better place?

What more could I want?
Clear as day, their forward movements

pushed into me and through me
with no stopping, and I felt their happiness.

A sensation then like those I remember
even now, of their being in utero;

I could feel them that autumn,
pushing themselves

forward into their lives,
all was right with the world.

So Far From Aloof

Only once in two-and-one-half years
did Lillian complain about going blind —
She needed to be somewhere without a ride
and could not drive, never did drive.
She said, *"the hand I am dealt"*
more than once.

When people first met Lillian, they
did not know she could not see them.
Her gaze direct, so far from aloof
yet, she worried friends thought she
was indifferent in public,
as she passed by.

Journal Entry – November 10, 2009
(Ten days before Lil was hospitalized)

While visiting Lillian at UNC this
past weekend, a first frost nailed
the nasturtiums and cosmos.
After two hours of pulling their
lifelessness out of the ground we
are left with Queen Ann's Lace,
alyssum, flowering Japanese
greens, and the magnificent blue-
green kale.

Now with the dead plants
removed, I look out at the side-
yard garden with a sense of
peace again.

I am learning to accept death,
using strength and will to clean up
what destruction comes,
sitting back to observe and
praise – and finding gratitude in
what is left living.

When even harder frosts strike,
I will look out, knowing seedlings
are safe under the cold frame
and hundreds of bulbs are
content to lay dormant, waiting
for spring.

I am flowing with the passage of
time, with life.

H-1-N-1

The first day of summer —
long hot glorious garden growing days.
Lillian rowed like a warrior, watched movies
and listened endlessly to her music
and took day trips to the beach
and ate pizza with girlfriends
wearing bright summer dresses
nails painted, hair put way up high.

Heat rolled in,
days lingered on
as H-1-N-1 bore down
on this unsuspecting country.

One daughter to head west
the other south. Logistics
overwhelming — but we got them there.
All was well. Continuous news flickering
this virus as we insulated into our lives.

Little did we know
the real life H-1-N-1 monster
would soon bore in and down
and explode into our precious
little one and take her,
just like that.

New Moon

One tiny candle pulsed from Lillian's
small half window. Hope emanated
large from that concrete gray building,
that hospital of miracles.

Patrick moved methodically
his large mass danced around her bed
working IV lines, replacing empty bags
hung from stalwart poles.

A liquid show of gravity forced
slow drips of meticulously
calculated pharmaceuticals,
into Lillian.

His 6'5" to her 5'2" —
he anointed her eyes and lips
to keep supple such sacred child
through the dark night,
that first Night of Lights.

I see him now, easily
lifting her in his arms
cradling her like an infant,
like a new life come to us

like the way
the new moon
holds the old moon
in its arms.

My Dear Lillian

You spin and whirl in your beautiful body full
of needles and tubes as big as garden hoses
that pump your blood out
into clear plastic for all
of us to see.

Eleven days cocktails of ammunition
have flowed through your veins.
When that war is over,
your body a battlefield
laid bare.

We wait for cool spring rains to push up
and out anything – tender and green.
Anything green. We wait
on sweet little miracles
rarely seen.

Your young woman body still beautiful
still strong, yet very still. We believe
there is time to win back
that precious body,
your life.

Instead my sweetheart, you are now our dance –
light music, toe tapping, soft shoeing,
spins and whirls, our dance always
ending in a dip followed forever,
over and over by our
endless ovation.

Viewing

Five o'clock am.
Here I am far
from the crowds

from strangers saying,
I am so sorry for your loss
followed by an attempt

to look deep
within my eye
hoping to see

a show of despair,
to witness a mother's
unraveling; this need

for drama, nothing more
than the worst
of human nature.

Shiva

Three nights ago we sat Shiva.
The kind rabbi running the show,
speaking ancient words for the community.

A scene acted out for the Jews of the family,
comforted while center stage – lights up,
standing room only, the lines spoken.

A playbill to take home,
to toss on the coffee table.

Five nights ago, at the viewing I raised my arms
to a thousand people come to see the mannequin
of my daughter. Crowds droned by, sprinkled
with dear friends and those unknown
drawn like magnets to my heart,
shocked into single grief.

At the end of the night, my body laden
with their hair and skin and essence –
a blanket of a heavy wet woolen humanity,
my center buried deep.

Like A Birthing

Ten days since our last kiss.
I removed tape from her face
to get at her sweet cheeks,
still warm.

One last embrace,
my arm haloed above her head
my head lightly on her chest.

A whispered farewell –
her ascent, while gravity
commanded me stay put.

Otis, what do we do now?

Whatever you say.

Turn off the machine.

The crank that made blood
that ran twenty-four seven/
twenty-three days
began to slow

Like a birthing –
only one direction,
Forward.
No turning back.

A Mortuary Tag

Attached to the left great toe,
an identification armband
  on the right wrist.

*"yes, make sure it is her
and no one else..."*

The body is that of a well developed
  well nourished young adult female.
63.5 inches.
Her scalp is covered with brown hair
  in a female pattern of distribution.
Irides are hazel in color, the pupils
  round, regular and equal.

*"63.5 inches, so carefully measured
her eyes are green, not hazel
be gentle, be gentle..."*

The nose unremarkable
  - external ears unremarkable.
  - teeth unremarkable.
  - tongue unremarkable.

*"Objection!
absolutely not possible!
this is too objective
even for death..."*

Identifying marks: none.

*"you simply did not look hard enough
impossible from the start."*

Inside Out

I feel crazy, like grief is gnawing away
    at me from the inside out,
like the carcass of that crow
    in the woods, over by North Lake

his eye intact, some feathers there
    and shiny with life.
Still, some of his bones are bare white
    half in/half out.

I do not want to get that far along
    and besides
I have not been left out in the elements,
    and I am still breathing.

Not once have I forgotten to breathe.

Sixteen Days Later

I marvel at my nails grown long
and my hair, no longer the shape I desire

I have stopped the urge
to trim everything back

Instead, I revel in
what has grown itself out.

A February Thanksgiving

Cleaning out the pantry
to find food for the crows
perched outside
screaming to be fed

Grabbing a bag of stuffing mix
and walking out through
the big-flaked February snow,
without thinking I crunch down
on a chunk of bread

The smell and tastes of Thanksgiving
blast through me –
instantly came
my family's favorite lost meal
in one blast of a bite

Memories of Thanksgiving 2009 –
Marching in a small circle
to the Macy's Day parade,
under the TV suspended from the wall
high up in Lillian's ICU cubical.

My parade and Lil's comments, a tradition –

*Mom insanely mimics whatever happens in the parade
and every year we laugh at her, and roll our eyes.*

And during the commercials
dinner gets cooked.

But on this February day,
seventeen previous
Thanksgivings tumble

through, in reverse order,
too many memories
too large to contain,

had the sage
not held it there.

Reminder Enough

Sometimes,
something so simple
as a wooden spoon
buried upright
in the coffee canister

bought in a lovely place,
in a kinder time

is reminder enough
for the stained mind
to reach beyond
the insistent pain, into
that next happy thing.

In The Rink

Less than two months
since Lillian's death
I am able to stand
on both feet longer,
a balance act –

the punches deeper
the belly bruised bluer
stains tattooed
one upon the other
no doubt,
a permanent thing.

Too Cruel to Oblige

I awoke willing the sun not to rise
wanting three more hours of dark,
wanting to stay put in my dreams

That place where seemingly
anything can relate to nothing.

A small hand
resting lightly on my shoulder,
urging me into the day where
wanting is no longer allowed.

Wanting wades one through hard waters
a lesson better quickly learned,
and for good.

Dreams are allowed, as are
vignettes of memories
both metered in short clips.

Allowed until driving pain
sees, and rips it all apart.

But wanting,
wanting – absolutely forbidden.

Drain yourself forever
of the smallest of wants:
            a cup of tea
                clothes cleaned
                    someone to say
                        the right thing.

For wanting the smallest of things
easily escalates into
wanting Lillian before me

And wanting Lillian before me
is an asking of this world
too cruel to oblige.

Brown Raincoat

The house empty as air,
Hannah and Eric on a four-day road trip
back to school. A bag stuffed and
left by the chair, I open to find
Lillian's brown raincoat.
Memories flood in –

She is a high school junior,
NYU and Columbia lure us to the City.
Lillian quickly dismisses both schools.

She realizes she cannot see
the subway map, her vision loss
constant, and gradual.

A champagne-colored dress hangs
at Loehmans in Chelsea
drastically reduced, her size zero.

She steps out of the dressing room.
A sweet, older sales lady all but screams,
My God, here is a Princess!

Within moments a clutch of employees
hands compulsively raised to their faces,
the dressing room turns magic.

They do not know their *Princess*
can not see them as she stands before
the mirror, that smile on her face.

The dress is purchased.

On the way out Lillian spots
a brown raincoat
and confesses she needs one.

This coat, now draped
over the corner of the bed,
very still. No longer needed.

Credulous

We humbly believe
we will go and
we will come again,
without fault.

Though we dangle
from this heavy test line,
hooks buried deep in the gill,
learn we must, to relax
into this weighty place.

Time

Please do not say time heals.
Time is a murderous thing.
The tic dulls and ages
her image, blurring
its edge.
There is no healing.

Time plays its nasty little role
each moment pushing away
her precious humanness,
retreating, as we helplessly
grasp our memories, unashamed.

Only fools who know no better
and know not their words
say *time heals* such a loss.

On my death day, Lil a fuzzy image,
an infectious chuckle, the shine and wave
of hair, a plump young cheek,
those eyes – that green,
will be with me, alive there
with me.

Comforting yet, still raw
a wound unhealed.
Time no healer,
time victorious.

A Half -Year Now

An old friend's familiar voice
screams out the message –

She wails over the phone,
begs forgiveness for not having known.

Where is my hole to burrow in,
to pry away summer's unbearable heat?

Today I want no one's sorrow laid raw.

I want only to make nestle like a mother

building walls around mid-afternoon,
finding sleep for her lost child

to watch moments tick
one more away,
so baby may slumber.

Game

Never has it been this long since I have not seen her, not since before her birth. I have not counted the days I have not seen her. I do not need to count the days I have not seen her because the tally is here, churning in my heart like an alarm that will not shut up. Not since before her birth have I gone so long without her voice or her image before me. Waiting to come upon her presence is a game that nobody wants to play, like playing Russian roulette, like knowing that you are in this game and you wonder how you could have ever agreed to this game, it's rules and regulations so unfair, so weighty, so inhuman, so serious: *"Game"* so ludicrously the wrong word for it. Like the word: "Life" … who imagined such words?

Family Dust

She left hair, flesh, and bones
behind and said

Do whatever with them.

We put them in a box
and put the box in the ground,
in a park of manicured beauty.

Still, dust balls of her hair
fly around the house,
particularly on the stairs

and in the heating vents.

Vacuuming,
a sacred event.

This Is The Girl

Who did not fall
into death's abyss.
She jumped,
deliberate – a diver
full of candor,
fearless

High up on a board
suspended, her
arms outstretched
knees pumping
up-and-down,
a willful act

Arching up
and then over,
her small hands together,
her feet pushed tight –
she leaps, an arrow
without aim

Falling away
from her fingers,
toes and hair – leaving
precious breath
and beat of heart
as senses shed.

So pure a scene that
at journey's end
her brilliance left
becomes for all,
an act surely we
aspire to follow.

All About

In this house
the cups and saucers stay in the cabinet
to the left of the sink

while our dear daughter
meanders through the woodwork and drapes,
and balances on the tips

of the cyclamen's upright petals,
and time demands backward while forward
struggles ahead

and sometimes she rests
there, serene in the sleepy half-closed
eyes of her two dogs.

Out the Door

Tilted toward autumn's
beginning, an energy rises
designed to nudge children
out the door and into a place
they call their own

We trust their new desk
suits them and their teachers care.
We pray they saddle up to the right kids
with an honest smile for that perfect
new friend

We moan summer's loss before
it has passed, while looking out
at dark cold, soon to bear down
as we dutifully believe the season
will bring them safely home.

The Next Empty Thing

Dear God,
Let me live with my altar hollow,
the kind of nothing that

talks about Lillian's body
out there
in the box

With no need
for one more glimpse
because one more

glimpse would be
just that —
nothing more.

Let the box and its contents
roll over into
that next empty thing.

She is now
what she always was
and always will be

far removed from sweet flesh
below earth's edge, and the image
in the yellow-framed picture.

She, with no script in hand
moves through us
She, the perfect actress

her words
confetti, tossed high
in the air.

Let Lillian be
her story, her story
enough.

Acknowledgements

My heartfelt thanks go to Dr. Fred Schiffman, who is the Sigal Family Professor of Humanistic Medicine at Alpert Medical School-Brown University. It was Dr. Schiffman who, in 2010, requested a compilation of poems to help medical students in the Gold's program learn about grief. Without his insistence and encouragement this little book would not exist.

Dr. Chuck Sherman and my husband, Eric Chason, likewise deserve thanks for their heartfelt, precious introductions to the poems as well as to our dear sweet Lillian.

Mary Pires has my gratitude for ploughing through an oversized shoebox of poems, scraps of writings, and journal entries to create the bones of this book. "This is what the medical students need to hear," she said.

Jill Culora was as efficient and smart as any editor I could have dreamed up. Thank you, Jill, for being there.

Brown University's hardworking, one-foot-out-the-door Gold Humanism Honor Society medical students deserve praise for bothering to read the poems and care about grief. They take my thanks with them as they head off to their residencies. We need these doctors in this world!

And lastly, I thank all the friends and strangers who contacted me over the last four years, asking when these poems would be put into print. Your generosity and caring have pushed me forward. The next book of poems will be for Non-Medical Students!